LIVER RESECTION SURGERY DIET

Empowering Your Healing Journey And Optimizing Recovery For Liver Health And Holistic Wellness

DR LUCAS KAYCE

DISCLAIMER

This book about illness and nutrition is not meant to replace expert medical advice, diagnosis, or treatment; rather, it is meant purely for informational reasons. This book's content is founded on broad concepts and recommendations for managing diseases and nutrition.

Before adopting any major dietary or lifestyle changes, readers are recommended to speak with a qualified healthcare provider, such as a licensed physician or registered dietitian, especially if they have pre-existing medical concerns. Everybody has different health demands, so what works for one person might not work for another.

The use of the information provided in this book may have unfavorable repercussions or consequences, for which the author and publisher disclaim all liability. No disease is meant to be identified, treated, cured, or prevented by the information provided.

The book may include contain references to medical literature or research findings; however readers are urged to independently confirm this material and contact reliable sources.

It is important to remember that the fields of nutrition and medicine are always changing, and that new findings could have an impact on the advice offered in this book. As a result, readers are urged to keep up with the most recent advancements in healthcare and, when in doubt, seek professional counsel.

By reading this book, readers agree that they are in charge of their own health decisions and release the author and publisher from any liability arising from the use of the material in the book, whether direct or indirect.

TABLE OF CONTENTS

ABOUT THE BOOK

One of the most important books on the subject of nutrition during the post-liver resection surgery healing process is The Liver Resection Surgery Diet. This book is important because it thoroughly examines the connection between food and the success of liver resection surgery. The book's goal is emphasized in the introduction, which also emphasizes how crucial a well-planned diet is to the process of rehabilitation as a whole.

The book explains the definition, goals, applications, risks, and benefits of liver resection surgery, providing a foundational understanding of the procedure. This background information gives readers a firm understanding of the surgical process and lays the groundwork for the sections that follow, which concentrate on the preoperative step. The significance of comprehensive preoperative planning, which includes lifestyle modifications and emotional preparedness, is emphasized throughout the book.

A large amount of the text is devoted to explaining the particular dietary guidelines that patients having liver resection surgery need to follow in advance of the treatment.

The relationship between diet and the healing process following surgery forms the central theme of the book. It clarify the critical role that nutrition plays in promoting the best possible recovery, highlighting the nutrients that are vital to the function of the liver, and providing dietary recommendations specific to candidates for liver resection. The book goes on to offer helpful advice on preoperative diet planning, including suggestions for foods high in protein, clear liquid diets, sources of carbohydrates, and vital vitamins.

As the book moves into the postoperative phase, it addresses pain and discomfort management, and continuous nutritional status monitoring, and methodically walks readers through the immediate and progressive diet progression. A thorough examination of special dietary considerations is provided, including adjustments for difficulties, methods for handling digestive problems, and ways to adjust for fluctuations in hunger.

Most importantly, the book broadens its focus to include long-term nutritional recommendations, stressing the creation of wholesome eating habits, avoiding weight swings, and continuously monitoring liver function through diet. The information supplied is made even more useful by the addition of nutrient-dense recipes, simple-to-make meal ideas, and cooking advice.

This book is a great resource for patients having liver resection surgery as well as the medical personnel who will be caring for them. Through its ability to connect the dots between dietary assistance and surgical intervention, it gives readers a comprehensive understanding and practical advice for a successful recovery.

DIET IS IMPORTANT FOR RECOVERY AFTER LIVER RESECTION SURGERY

It is impossible to overestimate the impact that diet plays in the healing process after liver resection surgery, as it promotes healing, reduces complications, and supports general well-being. Patients undergoing liver resection must follow a diet high in nutrients and balance because the liver is an important organ involved in many metabolic processes, such as digestion and nutrition absorption. After surgery, the nutrients obtained from food play a critical role in the liver's ability to heal and function at its best.

A piece of the liver is removed during liver resection surgery, which is sometimes required to cure diseases including tumors, cysts, or other abnormalities. During the critical postoperative phase, the body needs more resources to recuperate from the surgery and adjust to the altered shape and function of the liver. An important component of this healing process is an appropriate diet, which affects the patient's capacity to mend, restore strength, and avoid problems.

AN OVERVIEW OF SURGERY FOR LIVER RESECTION

A summary of liver resection surgery indicates that it is an intricate process requiring a thorough assessment of the patient's general condition, the degree of liver involvement, and any potential complications following the procedure. Depending on the particular medical situation, surgeons may remove the liver whole or in part. Although the liver has a remarkable ability for regeneration, the recuperation process can be taxing, requiring a multidisciplinary approach to patient care.

Following a liver resection, there are several different dietary factors to take into account. Enzyme and hormone synthesis, as well as tissue repair, depend on an adequate protein diet.

Lean protein foods including fish, chicken, and lentils are frequently recommended to patients. In addition, a balanced diet rich in lipids is vital for general health, while carbohydrates supply the energy required for recuperation. It's normal practice to closely monitor calorie intake to make sure patients are getting enough energy while preventing drastic weight loss.

In addition, being properly hydrated is crucial to the healing process. An appropriate fluid balance promotes the health of the organs and facilitates the body's removal of waste. During the early phases of recovery, patients are usually advised to maintain appropriate levels of hydration by drinking a combination of water, electrolyte-rich beverages, and, in certain situations, intravenous fluids.

Food affects more than just nutrition when it comes to liver resection surgery recovery; it also affects the body's inflammatory and immunological response. Fruits and vegetables are examples of foods high in antioxidants that are frequently advised to reduce oxidative stress and boost immunity. Furthermore, to maximize their recovery and long-term results, individuals with particular underlying conditions—such as diabetes or fatty liver disease—may need to make dietary alterations.

A good and uneventful postoperative course is contingent upon the role that diet plays in the recuperation process following liver resection surgery. A carefully thought-out and nutrient-dense diet promotes the patient's general health and resiliency in addition to helping the liver repair. The effectiveness of liver resection procedures depends more and more on a comprehensive approach to patient care that includes dietary advice as medical practitioners begin to identify the link between food and surgical results.

CHAPTER ONE

COMPREHENDING SURGERY FOR LIVER RESECTION

DEFINITION AND OBJECTIVE

Hepatectomy, or liver resection surgery, is a surgical technique used to remove part of the liver. The liver is an essential organ that performs several tasks, such as metabolism, detoxification, and the synthesis of proteins required for blood coagulation. Treatment for problems such as liver tumors, cysts, or other anomalies usually involves liver resection. The major goal of this procedure is to remove the damaged or diseased liver tissue while leaving the healthy tissue in place.

LIVER RESECTION TYPES

There are various kinds of liver resection procedures, and each is designed to meet the unique requirements of the patient. A partial hepatectomy, in which a portion of the liver is removed, is one frequent kind. When a localized tumor or lesion can be removed without impairing liver function as a whole, this treatment is frequently carried out. A total hepatectomy, in which the entire liver is removed, is an additional kind. This drastic procedure is, however, rarely used and is usually followed by a liver transplant.

REASONS TO REMOVE THE LIVER

For several disorders, liver resection is indicated, with the elimination of benign or malignant tumors being the main objective. hepatic resection may be indicated for hepatocellular carcinoma, hepatic hemangiomas, or metastatic liver tumors.

Patients with polycystic liver disease, liver cysts, or specific congenital defects affecting the structure of the liver may also benefit from this operation.

The choice to undergo a liver resection is carefully considered, taking into account the patient's general condition as well as the size, location, and kind of lesion.

Although liver resection surgery is a highly beneficial treatment option for liver problems, there are hazards associated with this procedure as well. Liver resection has the same risks as any surgical procedure: bleeding, infection, anesthesia-related complications. Furthermore, liver function may be impacted by liver resection, which could result in complications like liver failure. The liver can regenerate, though, and the healthy tissue that is still present can frequently make up for the function that has been lost, bringing the organ closer to its normal state over time.

Resection of the liver has many advantages, particularly in the case of cancer. Surgeons hope to eradicate cancerous cells and stop the disease from spreading by excising the affected portion of the liver. A successful liver resection can result in a substantial improvement in the general condition of the patient and, in certain situations, a full recovery. Furthermore, the process can reduce the symptoms of liver conditions that are not cancerous, giving affected individuals relief and enhancing their quality of life.

Liver resection surgery is a complex yet crucial procedure designed to treat various liver conditions by removing diseased or damaged tissue. The decision to undergo liver resection is carefully considered, taking into account the type and extent of the liver condition, as well as the overall health of the patient. While the surgery comes with inherent risks, the potential benefits, including the elimination of cancerous cells and improved liver function, make it a valuable option in the treatment of liver diseases.

CHAPTER TWO

PREPARING FOR LIVER RESECTION SURGERY

PREOPERATIVE ASSESSMENT

Before undergoing liver resection surgery, a thorough preoperative assessment is essential to ensure that the patient is in optimal health and prepared for the procedure. This assessment involves a comprehensive evaluation of the patient's medical history, current health status, and any pre-existing conditions.

The healthcare team will conduct various tests, including blood work, imaging studies, and cardiac evaluations, to assess the overall fitness of the patient for surgery.

This detailed assessment helps identify any potential risks or complications that may arise during or after the liver resection, allowing the medical team to tailor their approach and plan for a safe surgical procedure.

LIFESTYLE CHANGES BEFORE SURGERY

Making certain lifestyle changes before liver resection surgery is crucial to enhance the patient's overall well-being and improve the chances of a successful outcome. One of the primary considerations is the cessation of smoking, as smoking can impair lung function and hinder the body's ability to heal post-surgery. Additionally, patients are often advised to limit alcohol consumption to promote liver health and reduce the risk of complications. Engaging in regular physical activity, within the limits advised by the healthcare team, can also contribute to improved cardiovascular health and better postoperative recovery. These lifestyle adjustments are integral components of preoperative preparation, aiming to optimize the patient's condition for a smoother surgical experience.

EMOTIONAL PREPARATION

Preparing emotionally for liver resection surgery is an often overlooked but crucial aspect of the overall preoperative process. Facing major surgery can be emotionally challenging, and patients may experience anxiety, fear, or stress. Individuals must communicate openly with their healthcare providers about their emotional state, as this allows the medical team to provide necessary support and guidance. Engaging in discussions about the surgery, understanding the potential outcomes, and having realistic expectations can help alleviate emotional distress. Additionally, connecting with support groups, friends, or family members can provide valuable emotional support during this challenging time. Emotional preparedness is not only about understanding the medical aspects but also acknowledging and addressing the psychological impact of the impending surgery.

DIETARY CONSIDERATIONS BEFORE SURGERY

Proper dietary considerations before liver resection surgery play a vital role in promoting healing, reducing complications, and supporting overall recovery. Patients are typically advised to follow a well-balanced and nutritious diet in the weeks leading up to the surgery. This may include an emphasis on protein-rich foods to facilitate tissue repair and immune system function. Adequate hydration is essential to maintain optimal organ function and assist in the elimination of toxins from the body. Depending on the individual case, the healthcare team may recommend specific dietary restrictions, such as limiting fat intake or avoiding certain foods that could potentially impact liver function. Preoperative nutritional counseling is often provided to ensure that patients are well-informed and capable of making the necessary dietary adjustments to optimize their body's readiness for the upcoming liver resection surgery.

CHAPTER THREE

THE ROLE OF NUTRITION IN LIVER RESECTION SURGERY

IMPORTANCE OF NUTRITION IN SURGERY RECOVERY

The importance of nutrition in the context of liver resection surgery cannot be overstated, as it plays a crucial role in the overall recovery process. Adequate nutrition is vital for promoting wound healing, reducing the risk of infections, and supporting the body's ability to regenerate liver tissue.

Patients undergoing liver resection surgery often experience a significant metabolic demand due to the body's need for energy and nutrients to facilitate the healing process.

Therefore, a well-balanced and nutritionally rich diet is essential to enhance postoperative recovery and improve the patient's overall outcome.

NUTRIENTS ESSENTIAL FOR LIVER HEALTH

In the realm of liver health, specific nutrients play a pivotal role in supporting the functions of this vital organ. Proteins are fundamental for liver regeneration and repair, as they provide the necessary amino acids that contribute to tissue rebuilding. Additionally, amino acids aid in the synthesis of proteins essential for immune function, which is crucial in preventing postoperative infections. Omega-3 fatty acids, found in abundance in fatty fish, flaxseeds, and walnuts, have anti-inflammatory properties that can be beneficial for minimizing inflammation and promoting a healthy liver environment.

Vitamins and minerals also contribute significantly to liver health and recovery after surgery. Vitamin K, for instance, is essential for blood clotting, which is crucial in preventing excessive bleeding during and after surgery. B vitamins, particularly B12, and folate, play a role in red blood cell formation and overall energy metabolism.

Adequate intake of vitamin C supports collagen formation, contributing to the healing of surgical wounds. Minerals such as zinc and selenium are crucial for immune function and antioxidant defense, helping to protect the liver from oxidative stress.

DIETARY GUIDELINES FOR LIVER RESECTION CANDIDATES

For individuals undergoing liver resection surgery, adhering to specific dietary guidelines is imperative for optimizing outcomes. A diet rich in lean proteins, including poultry, fish, and legumes, ensures an adequate supply of amino acids essential for tissue repair. Incorporating a variety of fruits and vegetables provides essential vitamins, minerals, and antioxidants, promoting overall liver health. Monitoring and regulating fat intake, especially limiting saturated fats, can help manage inflammation and reduce the strain on the liver.

Hydration is another crucial aspect of postoperative nutrition. Staying adequately hydrated supports organ function and helps prevent complications such as constipation, which can be common after surgery. Maintaining a well-balanced diet that meets the nutritional needs of the individual patient is essential, and healthcare professionals often work closely with nutritionists to tailor dietary recommendations based on the patient's specific health status and surgical requirements.

The role of nutrition in liver resection surgery is multifaceted and paramount for the overall success of the procedure. A well-balanced diet that includes essential nutrients, vitamins, and minerals is crucial in promoting optimal recovery, reducing complications, and supporting the liver's regenerative capacity. Dietary guidelines tailored to liver resection candidates play a pivotal role in enhancing the postoperative journey and contributing to long-term liver health.

CHAPTER FOUR

PREOPERATIVE DIET PLANNING

CLEAR LIQUID DIET

A crucial aspect of preoperative diet planning is the implementation of a clear liquid diet. This dietary restriction involves consuming only transparent, liquid foods that leave minimal residue in the digestive tract. This is typically recommended in the immediate days leading up to surgery, aiming to ensure an empty stomach and reduce the risk of complications during the procedure. Clear liquids include water, broths, fruit juices without pulp, and clear gelatin. The goal is to provide hydration while minimizing the workload on the digestive system, thus facilitating a smoother surgical experience.

PROTEIN-RICH FOODS

Protein plays a vital role in the preoperative period, contributing to tissue repair and immune function. Incorporating protein-rich foods into the preoperative diet becomes imperative to optimize the patient's nutritional status. Sources such as lean meats, poultry, fish, eggs, dairy products, and plant-based options like legumes and tofu are essential. Adequate protein intake helps maintain muscle mass and supports the body's ability to heal post-surgery. This nutritional emphasis on protein is especially crucial for individuals undergoing major surgeries, as it aids in the recovery process and minimizes the risk of postoperative complications.

CARBOHYDRATES AND ENERGY SOURCES

Carbohydrates serve as a primary energy source for the body, making them a key component in preoperative diet planning. Consuming complex carbohydrates, such as whole grains, fruits, and vegetables, provides a sustained release of energy, aiding in the maintenance of blood glucose levels. This is particularly important to prevent fasting-induced hypoglycemia, which can negatively impact a patient's well-being before surgery. Balancing carbohydrate intake with other macronutrients ensures a steady energy supply, supporting the body's metabolic demands during the preoperative period and reducing the risk of complications related to energy depletion.

MICRONUTRIENT CONSIDERATIONS

Micronutrients, including vitamins and minerals, play a crucial role in supporting various physiological functions. In the preoperative context, ensuring adequate micronutrient intake is essential for optimizing the body's defenses and promoting healing. Vitamins such as vitamin C and vitamin A contribute to immune function and tissue repair, while minerals like zinc and iron play vital roles in wound healing and oxygen transport.

Incorporating a variety of colorful fruits and vegetables into the preoperative diet is a practical approach to obtaining a spectrum of micronutrients. However, caution should be exercised to avoid excessive intake of certain vitamins and minerals, as megadoses may interfere with the surgical process and postoperative recovery.

Preoperative diet planning involves a comprehensive consideration of various nutritional elements, each serving a specific purpose in preparing the body for surgery. The implementation of a clear liquid diet ensures a clean digestive system, while a focus on protein-rich foods, carbohydrates, and micronutrients contributes to overall nutritional optimization, supporting the body's resilience and facilitating a smoother recovery process post-surgery.

CHAPTER FIVE

POSTOPERATIVE NUTRITION AND RECOVERY

IMMEDIATE POSTOPERATIVE DIET

Postoperative nutrition plays a crucial role in the recovery process, with the immediate postoperative diet being a critical consideration. In the initial hours following surgery, patients are often advised to start with clear liquids to prevent dehydration and provide easily digestible nutrients.

This phase helps in easing the digestive system back into function while minimizing the risk of complications. As the patient tolerates clear liquids, the diet can progress to include more substantial options, such as broths and pureed foods.

GRADUAL PROGRESSION OF DIET

A gradual progression of the diet is essential to support the body's healing process. This involves advancing from liquids to soft and easily digestible foods, allowing the gastrointestinal system to gradually return to its normal function. This stepwise approach helps prevent postoperative complications, such as nausea and vomiting while ensuring that the patient receives the necessary nutrients for optimal recovery.

Healthcare professionals closely monitor the patient's tolerance and adjust the diet accordingly, ensuring a balance between providing nutrition and avoiding potential complications.

MANAGING PAIN AND DISCOMFORT

Managing pain and discomfort is an integral aspect of postoperative care, as pain can impact a patient's ability to eat and recover effectively. Adequate pain control measures, which may include medications or alternative therapies, play a crucial role in promoting appetite and facilitating the intake of essential nutrients.

Healthcare providers work closely with patients to tailor pain management strategies to individual needs, thereby enhancing overall postoperative recovery and nutritional intake.

MONITORING NUTRITIONAL STATUS

Monitoring nutritional status throughout the postoperative period is vital for assessing the patient's response to the diet and ensuring optimal recovery. Regular assessments include evaluating weight changes, nutritional intake, and any signs of malnutrition.

Blood tests may also be conducted to assess nutrient levels and identify deficiencies. This proactive approach allows healthcare professionals to identify and address any nutritional challenges promptly, supporting the patient's recovery and minimizing the risk of complications.

A comprehensive approach to postoperative nutrition and recovery involves an immediate postoperative diet that gradually progresses to more substantial options.

Managing pain and discomfort is crucial to facilitate proper nutrient intake, and constant monitoring of nutritional status ensures a proactive response to any challenges that may arise. By addressing these key concepts, healthcare providers can contribute to a smoother and more successful postoperative recovery for their patients.

CHAPTER SIX

PARTICULAR DIETARY REQUIREMENTS

DIETARY ADJUSTMENTS FOR PROBLEMS

One of the most important things to remember when dealing with specific dietary considerations is to adjust recipes to account for any difficulties that people may be experiencing. Tailored dietary programs are often necessary for several health issues, including diabetes, cardiovascular diseases, and renal disorders. For example, to properly control blood sugar levels, people with diabetes may need to keep an eye on how many carbohydrates they eat and prioritize meals with a low glycemic index. In a similar vein, people with heart problems could find that eating less sodium and saturated fats helps maintain heart health.

Adjustments are necessary when there are certain dietary restrictions or allergies to avoid negative effects. For example, people with celiac disease require a gluten-free diet since they must strictly avoid foods that contain gluten. Customizing the diet to deal with issues not only helps with disease management but also improves general health.

HANDLING INTESTINAL PROBLEMS

A person's diet and way of life can be greatly impacted by digestive problems. Meal planning needs to take into account medical conditions such as lactose intolerance, Crohn's disease, and irritable bowel syndrome (IBS). In certain situations, an IBS sufferer may be advised to follow a low-FODMAP diet that focuses on avoiding specific fermentable carbs that may exacerbate symptoms. A diet low in fiber and easily digested during flare-ups may be helpful for those with Crohn's disease.

To minimize stomach pain, those with lactose sensitivity must avoid dairy products or utilize lactose-free alternatives. It is crucial to speak with medical specialists or registered dietitians when managing digestive problems to develop a customized strategy that takes care of certain symptoms and encourages good digestion.

ADJUSTING TO MODIFICATIONS IN HUNGER

Numerous variables, such as aging, medical treatments, or psychological problems, can be responsible for changes in appetite. Chemotherapy patients, for example, may lose their appetite or develop new taste preferences. I

n these situations, modifying the diet to account for these modifications is essential to guarantee sufficient nourishment and avoid malnourishment.

It can be beneficial to adjust meal plans to accommodate people with different taste preferences or to spread out smaller, higher-nutrient meals throughout the day. Anger or sadness are examples of psychological variables that might affect hunger.

In such cases, emphasizing nutrient-dense foods and seeking advice from dietitians or mental health specialists might help in formulating plans to address the nutritional and psychological components of hunger fluctuations.

Specific dietary concerns cover a wide range of topics, such as adjustments for difficulties, handling of digestive problems, and flexibility in response to fluctuations in hunger. Tailoring dietary programs to meet the specific needs of each person facing a particular difficulty can help to improve overall well-being, optimize health, and control symptoms.

CHAPTER SEVEN

CREATING A BALANCED DIETARY SCHEDULE

Sustaining a nutritious diet is essential for general health and long-term well-being. This entails choosing wholesome foods as well as creating a regular, balanced eating schedule. Including a range of food groups is essential, including whole grains, fruits, vegetables, lean meats, dairy products, and dairy substitutes. Maintaining equilibrium between these components guarantees that the body gets the nutrition it needs, enabling the best possible performance of numerous physiological functions.

Furthermore, maintaining a consistent meal schedule helps to stabilize blood sugar levels and discourage unhealthy snacking, which promotes a long-term nutritional plan. Establishing a healthy eating regimen can also be greatly aided by meal planning ahead of time and mindful eating techniques. People can improve their digestion and nutrient absorption by cultivating a thoughtful relationship with food by being attentive to portion amounts and savoring every bite.

PREVENTING WEIGHT GAIN AND LOSS

A comprehensive strategy that goes beyond fad diets or drastic measures is needed to maintain a healthy weight, which is the cornerstone of long-term dietary guidelines. Preventing weight gain and reduction requires a mix of a conscious eating style, frequent exercise, and a well-balanced diet. A healthy weight is easier to reach and maintain when nutrient-dense foods are prioritized and processed and high-calorie foods are consumed in moderation.

Frequent exercise helps you burn calories and improves your general health, which makes it an essential part of weight management. A complete strategy for weight maintenance includes a combination of strength training, flexibility exercises, and cardiovascular activities.

Furthermore, minimizing unhealthful weight fluctuations requires developing a good body image and a balanced relationship with food, which emphasizes the need for self-care and mental health.

KEEPING AN EYE ON LIVER HEALTH WITH FOOD

The liver is essential to detoxification, metabolism, and general health. It is imperative to monitor liver health through dietary decisions to promote normal liver function and prevent illnesses such as fatty liver disease. Preventing the build-up of fat in the liver requires limiting the consumption of processed foods, refined carbohydrates, and saturated fats. Rather, by supplying vital nutrients and antioxidants, a diet high in fruits, vegetables, whole grains, and lean meats promotes liver function.

Another important component of preserving liver health is staying hydrated since water helps the body eliminate toxins and supports healthy liver function. Coffee consumption in moderation, which has been linked to liver-protective qualities, might also be taken into account. Including foods high in chemicals that are beneficial to the liver, such as garlic, turmeric, and cruciferous vegetables, regularly supports the health of this important organ. Individualized advice on preserving liver health through food selections can be obtained through routine examinations and meetings with medical specialists.

CHAPTER EIGHT

RECIPES FOR RECOVERING AFTER LIVER RESECTION

RICH IN NUTRIENT RECIPES

Choosing nutrient-dense dishes is important since they offer vital vitamins, minerals, and other nutrients to aid in the healing process after liver resection. A well-rounded and balanced diet is ensured by including a range of colorful vegetables, lean proteins, and healthy grains. Take into account recipes that highlight foods high in antioxidants, such as cruciferous vegetables, berries, and leafy greens, which can aid in liver health and inflammation reduction.

Lean proteins, such as chicken, fish, and tofu, can help with tissue repair and muscle maintenance in addition to veggies. Pick dishes that include almonds, avocados, and olive oil—sources of healthy fats—to enhance energy levels and the body's overall ability to absorb nutrients.

It's critical to concentrate on a wide variety of nutrient-dense foods to provide the body with the building blocks it needs to heal.

SIMPLE-TO-COMB

Dinner Ideas Choosing simple meal ideas are essential for a more seamless recovery process because of the possible difficulties with digestion following liver resection. When compared to their raw counterparts, cooked vegetables—like steamed carrots or mashed sweet potatoes—are easier on the digestive tract. In a similar vein, including well-cooked grains such as quinoa or rice can supply energy without overtaxing the digestive system.

Select simple-to-digest lean proteins, like grilled or poached chicken, and think about adding plant-based protein sources, like soft tofu or lentils. Making soups and stews with nutrient-dense ingredients may be soothing for the body and gentle on the stomach. Incorporating readily digestible fruits, such as cooked apples or bananas, can sate sweet tooths without taxing the digestive system.

RECIPES FOR A HEALED LIVER

It's critical to follow cooking guidelines that put liver health first while preparing meals for liver resection rehabilitation. To maintain a healthy liver, consuming too few fats overall—especially saturated and trans fats—is essential. Instead of frying, use cooking techniques like baking, grilling, or steaming, which retain food's nutritious value without adding extra fat.

When it comes to salt consumption, moderation is essential because too much sodium can cause fluid retention and even strain the liver. It makes sense to use herbs and spices to provide flavor instead of salt. Since water-rich vegetables like cucumbers and watermelon are essential for liver function, including them in your diet will help you consume more fluids overall.

A careful approach to nutrient-dense meals, simple-to-digest meal ideas, and cooking advice that is favorable to the liver can greatly aid in a good recovery following liver resection. Customizing the diet to each person's tastes and tolerances is crucial, but the main goal should always be to support and encourage liver function and promote healing.

CHAPTER NINE
MODIFICATIONS TO LIFESTYLE FOR LONG-TERM LIVER HEALTH

EXERCISE SUGGESTIONS

Adopting a comprehensive strategy that includes numerous lifestyle adjustments is necessary to ensure long-term liver health. Physical activity regularly is essential. Exercise is very important for liver health in addition to being a great way to maintain general well-being. Exercise improves blood flow, which supports the liver's effective operation. Additionally, it aids in weight management and the prevention of diseases like non-alcoholic fatty liver disease (NAFLD), a prevalent liver ailment linked to obesity.

STRESS REDUCTION

Another essential element of preserving the best possible liver health is stress management. Prolonged stress can negatively impact the liver, exacerbating inflammation and other conditions linked to the liver. Stress reduction methods that work well include deep breathing techniques, mindfulness, and meditation. Long-term liver health protection and stress management include establishing a good work-life balance, including leisure activities, and getting emotional support.

AVERTING DANGEROUS SUBSTANCE USE

Steer clear of dangerous chemicals if you want to keep your liver healthy. Reducing alcohol intake is essential since heavy drinking might cause diseases like alcoholic liver disease. For those with pre-existing liver diseases, it is best to follow prescribed alcohol intake guidelines or refrain from alcohol entirely. Prescription drugs and illegal drugs should also be avoided as they may have harmful effects on the liver. It is essential to regularly check drug use under the supervision of medical specialists to avoid potential liver damage.

Long-term liver health is also significantly influenced by dietary practices. Optimizing liver function can be achieved through eating a well-balanced diet high in fruits, vegetables, whole grains, and lean proteins. A few meals, such as those high in antioxidants and anti-inflammatory qualities, can help shield the liver from harm. Maintaining adequate hydration is also crucial since it helps the liver operate by aiding in the detoxification process.

Another important strategy for long-term liver health promotion is maintaining a healthy body weight. Obesity can worsen pre-existing liver disorders and is strongly associated with the development of fatty liver disease.

Preventing issues connected to liver disease requires implementing a balanced and sustainable strategy for weight control through a combination of regular exercise and a healthy diet.

Maintaining long-term liver health requires embracing a lifestyle that places a high priority on consistent exercise, efficient stress management, and abstaining from dangerous substances.

These all-encompassing adjustments support mental and physical wellness in addition to liver health. Long-term quality of life can be improved and the risk of liver-related disorders can be considerably decreased by making educated decisions in daily life.